IF YOU ARE WHAT YOU EAT, SHOULD I EAT A SKINNY GIRL?

TIPS AND ADVICE ABOUT LOSING THE WEIGHT
WITHOUT LOSING YOUR APPETITE FOR LIFE

NATHALIE BOTROS
THE Bon-Vivant girl

If You Are What You Eat, Should I Eat a Skinny Girl?
Tips and Advice For Losing the Weight But Not Your Appetite For Life

Publisher: The Bon-Vivant Girl

Cover Design: Mark Duebner Design

The content of this book is for general instruction only. Each person's physical, emotional, and spiritual condition is unique. The instruction in this book is not intended to replace or interrupt the reader's relationship with a physician or other professional. Please consult your doctor for matters pertaining to your specific health and diet.

ISBN-10: 0-9985512-0-1

ISBN-13: 978-0-9985512-0-3

Printed in the United States of America

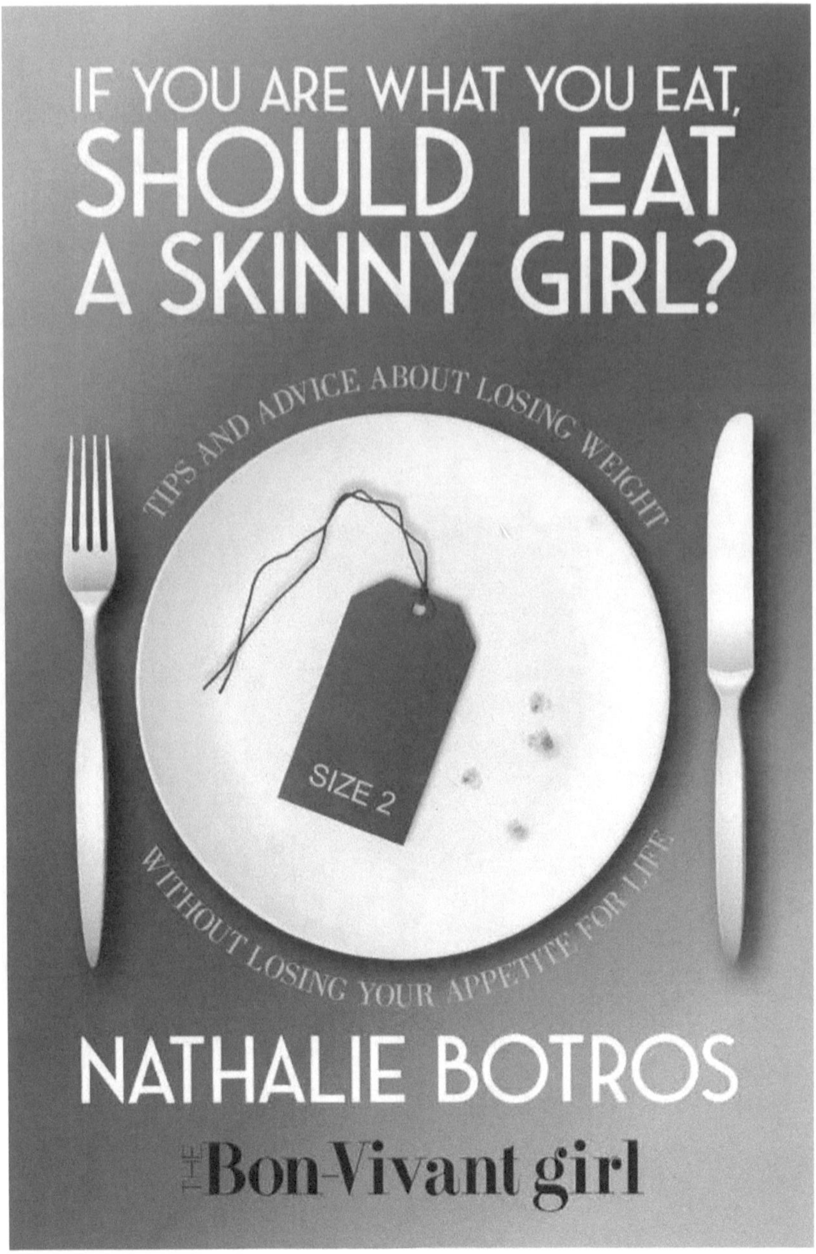
IF YOU ARE WHAT YOU EAT,
SHOULD I EAT
A SKINNY GIRL?
TIPS AND ADVICE ABOUT LOSING WEIGHT
SIZE 2
WITHOUT LOSING YOUR APPETITE FOR LIFE
NATHALIE BOTROS
THE Bon-Vivant girl

CONTENTS

To my queen mom, my sis,

and to all the bon-vivant girls.

INTRODUCTION

Every woman I know has a problem with her body. Too short, too tall, too ugly, too skinny (yes, it does exist), and the infamous too fat.

I am not an exception, I have struggled with my weight all my life.

Is it genetic? Probably, because all my family struggles with the same problem.

Is it cultural? Probably as well, because my mom always taught me to finish my plate and never say no to a second serving. She said it was rude to say no.

I can come up with so many excuses, and I know you all can too. We all have legitimate reasons for why we have some pounds to shed or why we gained weight.

Does that mean we should accept our gained weight? No!

Does that mean we should dedicate our lives to losing weight? Definitely not!!!

Let's be honest, at the end of the day, our extra weight didn't creep in overnight and attack us. We gained it through our choices.

While there are some things that I cannot change about my body, like my height or my bone structure, what I can do is change my way of thinking, accept my body, and work on myself.

So can you.

ON THE CONTRARY TO WHEN PEOPLE SAY, "YOU ARE WHAT YOU EAT," YOU SHOULDN'T NEED TO EAT A SKINNY PERSON TO BE SKINNY.

Some can say I am a party girl, some a jetsetter. I would consider myself more a "bon vivant" who enjoys every minute of life. I was born in Lebanon, raised in Switzerland, and have lived in Turkey and Europe before moving to New York a couple of years ago. I am lucky enough to travel all around the world, to see amazing things, and to eat at delicious restaurants with the best chefs.

I started dieting when I was fourteen years old because everyone was doing it. I was in boarding school in Switzerland—you know, the paradise of chocolate and cheese. I remember my first diet consisted of eating only apples and yogurt just before going home. I would lose a few pounds, and the minute I arrived home, I gained them back eating my mom's delicious dishes.

My diets varied depending on where I lived and what was "the little black dress of diets" at the time. I had to follow the fashion. Over the course of my life, I have tried hundreds of diets. Name the diet and I've tried it. Low carb, high protein, South Beach, holistic, vegetarian, rice, juicing... I have even injected myself with pregnancy hormones. I've tried all the diet pills, acupuncture, cupping... again, name it and I've tried it. I've even had liposuction.

Some of those diets helped me lose weight. Although, as soon as I finished the diet, I thought I was invincible and started to eat the way I used to. And guess what? I gained back the weight and even added a few more pounds because I didn't learn how to eat right. I just put my body into restriction for a while.

Does any of this ring a bell?

I made another common mistake. I listened to every commercial and every friend around me about whatever diet worked for them. Guess what? Every diet is not suitable for everyone!

I managed to find a balance with my weight and diets, but when I moved to NY, things changed. I don't know if it was the constant food TV adds, the junk food world, or the easy food deliveries, but I gained more than forty pounds without noticing. Again, I can blame everything and anything, but at the end of the day, I ate that food to gain weight.

I felt fat, and would sit in front of my closet every day and cry.

You know when you gain a few pounds, your pants get tighter? Well, my wardrobe was six sizes tighter.

Panicked and desperate, I dedicated my life to losing weight. I stopped traveling, stopped eating out. I became obsessed with diets and exercise. I followed what people proposed: "If you want to lose weight, eat less and start working out." I started working out. I did an hour of cardio five days a week, Pilates three times a week, and I worked with a personal trainer twice a week. I also adopted a strict diet. On top of it all, I got regular massages.

The result? Besides having a hole in my pocket, I had strong abs surrounded by fat, and I looked like a catcher because I'd gained muscle without losing any weight. Sexy, right? On top of it all, I was unhappy, with no social life.

I thought something was wrong with me. I took all the medical tests available—checked my thyroid, my blood, everything. I was in perfect health.

What was I doing wrong???

If you are reading this book, it means all of this reminds you of yourself. You did all the right things, yet you still cannot lose weight. After years of struggling, I have noticed something. You can do everything right, but if you are not doing it with joy and you are not happy with your life, it won't work.

I know that when we gain weight, we are not happy about ourselves and our bodies. Although, I learned something during my journey. Losing weight is not going to make you happier. If that theory were correct, every skinny person in this world should be happy!

You won't be happier if you are skinny. Don't think that your life is going to change and everything is going to be peachy because you lost a few pounds.

Although it looks like we're not motivated because the weight won't go away, and people judge us about our efforts, I understand that you're desperate. I was desperate too. Remember, I injected myself with pregnancy hormones. I think when you come to the point of stabbing yourself with a needle or starving yourself just to lose few pounds, one can call it desperate and motivated.

So, why we are not shedding the extra weight?

Because we are using the wrong solution to the problem. We are "serial dieters" and restricting ourselves from living. When I came to that conclusion, I decided no more diets for me. I needed a new lifestyle.

It took me some time to get there. I needed to work on myself first.

During that period, I had highs and lows with my weight. This time, I didn't panic when I gained few pounds. Instead, I had to study myself. The key was to understand why I gained that weight. Was it emotional or simply a hungry period? Studying my weight gain helped me to resolve that issue. For example, I know that when I have family or friends visiting, I automatically eat more, as everybody is hungry at different hours.

My resolution was to be a bit more careful with food before their visits so I could earn "food credits." Thanks to my food credits, I can enjoy food when family and friends are around.

I also want you to understand that PERFECT doesn't exist. Why do you think John Knoll created Photoshop? It is to cut, add, and reshape a real woman's body into an unreal person. Guess what? Even the women that you see in magazines are not perfect and not happier than you. I know a lot of models, and those women that you idealize on magazines are not real. They have been photoshopped. On top of it, even they complain about their bodies.

Unfortunately, in the world today, all the magazines give us a wrong picture of the perfect body image. They make us believe that if we look like "hangers," we are perfect. You are a woman.

> EMBRACE YOUR CURVES AND SHAPES. EVERYTHING STARTS WITH YOU. IF YOU LOVE THEM, THEN OTHERS WON'T HAVE ANY OTHER CHOICE BUT TO LOVE THEM.

Today, I am in the best shape of my life.

Am I skinny like a model? No.

Am I fat? No.

Am I healthy and happy? Yesss.

My friends and family cannot believe my transformation. They keep asking me, "How can you have a social life, go out, travel, and keep the weight off? Could you tell me your diet?" My answer is: I am done with diets. I propose a new lifestyle.

I am dedicating this book to all the bon-vivant girls out there who are hiding because they don't feel good in their skin. I am not proposing you another diet. I am showing you that you can have a glamorous and social life while being healthy, and still lose weight. It is just about changing a few habits.

Is it going to be easy every day? Of course not. Is it worth it?

Damn yes.

One

IF YOU ARE WHAT YOU EAT, SHOULD I EAT A SKINNY GIRL? (TIPS AND ADVICE ABOUT HOW TO START YOUR JOURNEY)

1. Love Yourself and Accept Your Body.

I know it sounds cheesy, and if someone had told me that years ago, I would've laughed in their face and said, "Really? Come on, hippie."

Also, you might think, "If I love myself and my body, why should I lose weight?"

The reason is simple. To be able to achieve anything, you need to accept the situation first. Once you accept your body, you can move forward.

So, basically, follow Mr. Darcy's key sentence, "Like yourself just the way you are."

I remember, I had just started dating this guy and I thought he would see that I was chubby right away. I thought it was smart to let him know why I had a few extra pounds and started telling him my story about how I'd gained weight the last few years. He looked at me and said, "Oh, I didn't notice you had weight to lose," and started to look at me differently. He didn't even notice my extra weight, until I pointed out.

We must accept who we are and love ourselves to achieve anything. How do you expect your body to respond if you hate it? Whether you've gained three, ten or forty pounds, it is still your body and you must love it.

Don't forget: Every extra pound is extra of you to love.

Kubler-Ross created five stages of grief and loss for when we lose someone we love. Why don't we use that to grieve and accept our new forms? Because the key to a healthier and skinnier life is to accept and love who we are.

DENIAL

The denial stage is the beginning. You don't want to accept that you gained all that weight. You always blame other factors. Your clothes got smaller because of the dry cleaner or because you put them in the dryer. During that period, I think I changed three dry cleaners.

Once, when I had to attend a wedding in Lake Como, I insisted on bringing my old evening gown from the time I used to be lighter. The day of the wedding, obviously, the zipper wouldn't go up. So, I had to be creative at the last minute and wear a jacket on top so no one would see that the dress was open in the back. Let me tell you, with the heat of summer and that jacket, I was melting.

We all have great excuses rooted in denial. The one that I love is when you cannot close your pants and say, "I am bloated today." Honey, you have been bloated for the past ten years. Wake up!!!

I have started to avoid things that would make me fat: scales, mirrors, and photos.

ANGER

My denial turned into anger.

Needless to say, I was first angry at myself: How did I get here?!? I knew the clothes were tight and that I'd gained weight, but instead of looking at my eating habits, I was angry at everyone and everything. You can ask my mother and my sister—I constantly snapped at them.

With my friends, I express my anger silently. I used to sit at the table with a smile, and judge every bite of food they ate. I thought it was unfair. Why me? How come they eat more than I do and they are thinner?

And of course, I was angry at my scale, my dry cleaner, and my dryer for letting me down.

I put my scale in the corner of the bathroom and told it, "You won't come out from there until you show me good results."

BARGAINING

During the bargaining stage, I accepted I had a weight problem, but then started looking for a simple way to get out of it.

The first step was to bargain with a higher power than myself. GOD. I kept asking God to help me lose weight.

When that didn't work, I moved on to step two.

What if I cut all carbs, protein, or white food from my life? Will I be skinny again?

Then, once I had tried all the possible diets on the market with no success, my ultimate bargaining pitch became, "If I put myself in the dryer or send myself to the dry cleaner, will I shrink like my clothes?"

DEPRESSION

At this point, I knew I had gained the weight and neither anger nor bargaining would help me. Life was sad. I tried everything, and still no results. I sat in front of my closet with tears in my eyes, trying to find something to wear.

I thought that everybody could only see "the fat chick" in me. That feeling made me stop wanting to go out and socialize. I would spend my days home, feeling sorry for myself. You know the feeling when you hit rock bottom, where nothing seems to be a solution.

Some people stop eating when they are depressed. I belong to the other category—I eat my feelings.

You know how when you are depressed, you try to find your happy place? Well, my happy place was the fridge.

ACCEPTANCE

Halleluiah!!! The day came when I accepted my body, and I was ready to move on. This person is who I am right now, and I will change it. Suddenly a huge weight was lifted from me—not on the scale, but off my mind.

My acceptance was thanks to a TV show.

One day, depressed in front of my TV, I watched a show called How to Look Good Naked in which a fashion stylist encourages women who are insecure with their bodies to strip nude for the camera. He builds the women's self-esteem by helping them to shop and to dress. In the final scene, he displays the women's pictures in a public place and asks passerby's their opinion. As the response is always positive, the women build a higher self-esteem.

Evidently, I didn't participate in the show, and didn't put my naked picture on a billboard, but it made me think. When we gain weight, we feel fat and ugly. No matter what outfit we put on, we see all our flaws. I remember thinking that I looked like a monster.

I DECIDED TO BREAK THE CYCLE AND AT LEAST LOVE ONE THING ABOUT MY BODY EVERY WEEK.

So, for weeks, I stood naked in front of my mirror and learned to like my body and accept my new forms.

You know when they say, "Fake it until you make it?" Well, I did it, and decided that I was hot and voluptuous. My friends would say, "You look so much more at peace with yourself that no one would even dare to say that you need to lose weight."

My second step was to go out and shop for the right size clothes. I didn't buy a lot; just a few essential pieces—a black pant, few black tops, and a lot of accessories. Guess what? On my scale, I was the same weight, but people started asking me if I had lost weight.

I can say that was the first step of my new life.

2. Don't Ever Think You Are on a Diet. This is a Lifestyle.

Have you ever Googled the definition of "diet?" I did it for you: "A special course of food to which one restricts oneself, either to lose weight or for medical reasons."

Who wants to be restricted? When we say, "I am on a diet," we get instantly hungry and start cheating. Don't use that word. Say, "I am on a health kick," or, "...my new lifestyle." It won't have the same connotation of punishment.

I don't want you to end up writing a breakup letter to dieting:

Dear diet,
Things are not going well between us. You are boring, and I keep cheating on you...

A friend once mentioned to me, "We have to accept that some people like us always have tendencies to gain weight. So, we have to be careful with what we eat all the time."

Does that mean I need to be on a "diet" my whole life? Hell no. No one wants to or can say they are on a diet their whole life, so let's call it our new "lifestyle."

3. Don't Believe in Friends, Magazines, or TV Diets. Each Person is Different.

Some people eat to live. I live to eat.

Even when I am eating at a restaurant, I talk about other foods and restaurants. Talking about food leads to the conversation of diets. We all have friends who tell us "how to lose the weight." Stop listening to friends, TV, and books. Listen to yourself.

You know what is right for you and what is bad for you.

Everybody has a theory, but don't forget that a diet that worked for a friend could be terrible for you. The reason is simple. First, each person's constitution is different. We have different shapes and genetics, so each person works differently. Some people burn calories just by sitting in front of the TV; others lose the calories by working out long hours. We have different lifestyles. Some of us spend our days in front of a computer; others spend their days running around from meeting to meeting. How can we expect that the same diet will work the same way for everyone?

For example, if I restrict my calories, I can shed a few pounds. I know that it is not a lifelong solution, but it works in the short-term. However, I've advised friends to do this in the past and it was a catastrophe for them, as they got tired counting every bite.

Tell me if these sentences make sense to you:

"Oh, did you see that commercial on TV? You can lose ten pounds in two weeks with this supplement. And you can still eat whatever you want."

Let me tell about that commercial. Among a hundred people, it maybe worked on two. The reality is that you are taking a supplement that is full of chemicals. Sure, it may make you lose ten pounds in ten days, but what about the eleventh day when you put five pounds back on??

"My friend, Jessica, lost twenty pounds when she became vegan."

I respect everybody's choice, but I personally cannot conceive of life to be all about ruminating vegetables. I have tried the vegetarian diet, and I was "Mrs. Fartalot," with a big tummy because of all those fibers. People would ask me when I was due. I would answer them, "Any time now, but you should step back..."

You will always hear about those diets—some magic, some real, it can work on your friends for a while, but it doesn't mean it will work for you. So how to choose what works for you? Simply by studying yourself with your food journal.

4. *Create a Food Journal.*

Besides getting ready psychologically, you need to get ready practically as well.

Before you start your journey, I would like you to write down everything you eat for a week, even the little cookie you took from your kid's snack or the three olives that you ate while cooking.

Don't lie, be honest. No one is judging you.

We all say, "I didn't eat anything today. How come I gained weight?" Well, what about the five crackers, two cheese slices, and the cold cuts while you cooked? Just because you didn't sit and eat it, doesn't mean it doesn't count!!!

In your food journal, you should add the food, the time, and the quantities. Create a column where you write where are you when you eat these things and what are you doing. Create another column where you put your mood.

Now, you cannot always fill up the mood column, but try to describe how you feel before, after, and while you are eating. With time, you can log even more info, like how much water you drank during the day or your workouts.

Your food journal could look like the example on the next page:

TIME	FOOD	WHERE/WHY	MOOD
6am	*wheat flake cereal with milk and 1 banana*	*home/ breakfast*	*tired*
7am			
8am			
9am	*coffee*	*office*	
10am			
11am	*kale salad with chicken, whole wheat bread*	*office lunch*	*hungry*
12pm			
1pm	*coffee*		
2pm			
3pm			
4pm	*a bite of chocolate bar*	*office/shared my colleague's*	*because it was there*
5pm			
6pm			
7pm	*3 cheese slices, 2 olives*	*home/while cooking*	
8pm	*baked salmon with spinach*	*home/dinner*	
9pm	*3 chocolate cookies*	*home/washing clothes*	
10pm			
11pm	*popcorn*	*home/ watching TV*	*bored*
12pm			

5. Become Your Own Nutritionist: How to Read and Interpret Your Food Journal.

Once you've finished with your journal at the end of the week, answer these questions:

- What are my bad and good foods?
- When am I the hungriest? Breakfast, lunch, dinner, or even at 4 pm? Why?
- When and what do I crave? Study your cravings.
- Why do I have those cravings? Because of hunger or a particular time or after a life event?
- What are my quantities?

You can already see what's wrong and what's right. You don't need to see a nutritionist or to follow a strict diet. Just view yourself as a case study, and see what you can do with your "wrongs."

BAD FOOD VERSUS GOOD FOOD

When you read your food journal, you can already see what your weak and healthy foods are.

For example, I know my weakness is cheese. I am capable of eating a shoe sole if you melt cheese on it.

So, already decreasing the amount of cheese will help me shed a few pounds. I am saying reduce, not CUT. I don't want to feel deprived. But when I shop, I never buy a lot of cheese anymore.

If it is not in my fridge, I cannot eat it.

WHEN AM I THE HUNGRIEST? DEFINE THE DANGEROUS HOUR.

We all know when we are the hungriest. Some people wake up hungry. Some people, like me, are not hungry until 1 or even 2pm.

I know everyone says the most important meal of the day is breakfast. I don't agree. If I am not hungry, why I should eat? I think the most important meal of the day depends on your life, work, and personality.

Some people are hungry when they come home from work, so they eat a whole meal and then eat dinner.

Some people feel famished after dinner—as we call it, "the night snacking." You have been good all day. At night, you eat your healthy dinner and start watching TV. Then, you don't know if it is due to constant food advertisements, your motionless body, or simply boredom, but at some point, you feel like nibbling on something. You try to resist, drink water, and tell yourself, "Forget about it." The more you try to forget, the more it becomes an obsession, and the kitchen is calling for you. You finally make the move. You can hear voices telling you, like in horror movies, "Don't go there. Don't open that door," and you imagine the calories like little devils waiting behind the door. Of course, you do open the door and eat a salty snack, then crave for a sweet snack... and just like in every horror movie, your end isn't a happy one. You feel guilty and fat.

How can you avoid this? Have good snacks ready to eat. We will talk more about it in the coming chapters.

CRAVINGS

We all have cravings. They can be savory, sweet, or both. With your food journal, you can already pinpoint when and what you crave. Again, study and analyze yourself.

Is it right after work when you arrive home or at 7pm? Why? It might be because you didn't have time for lunch, in which case it makes sense that you are hungry. Although, no one told you to starve yourself. Another reason could be that when you come home, you need to unwind with food. This describes expressing your emotions with food.

If it is emotional eating, you are the only one who will know why. Try to figure out the reasons. Problems with work? Relationship? Or just boredom? You have the tools to conquer. I believe in you.

My cravings are always late at night when I am home, watching TV. I always feel like eating something salty. Then, it is too salty, so I crave sweet. With time, I noticed that I had those cravings because I was bored and would fill the boredom with food. When I am out, I don't have the same problem, as I am busy talking with people and socializing. So, what to do? I cannot be out every night!!!

I decided to keep myself busy. Instead of watching TV as if I am lobotomized, I keep myself busy with different tasks. My favorite is catching up on the ones that I keep postponing, like organizing my address book on my PC or phone. It resolves several problems at the same time—too busy to have cravings, and a painful job gets done.

I found my solution while I was studying myself. You should do the same.

I know that you will need time to resolve your cravings, so the immediate solution is to drink a glass of water and wait half an hour. Still craving? Drink another glass... Just kidding. If the hunger persists, eat your prepared snack. Make sure to have sweet and savory snacks so that you can satisfy the correct craving.

QUANTITIES

To log your quantity of food in your journal is essential. Sometimes we don't eat a variety of food categories, but we eat a lot. We might think we didn't eat a lot as we don't even notice how much we eat. So, writing down the quantity will show us if we ate a lot or not enough.

I personally know that one of my big mistakes was quantities. With reducing portion sizes and varying food categories, I noticed that I was less hungry and that I have lost weight.

6. Don't Believe You Will Lose Weight in Three Days. It Took You Years to Gain It.

Another important thing is to not fall into fad diets.

Honey, you haven't gained this weight overnight, so don't expect to lose it in three days. Of course, if you starve yourself, you will lose few pounds in three days. These lost pounds won't be the fat, but water.

I know it is easier to think that we haven't done anything wrong, and like little nasty creatures, the weight attacked us overnight. I wish that was true, but unfortunately, it is not. We gained that weight over time. I am not talking about the two pounds that you gained from last night's dinner because you ate very salty Chinese food and you have water retention. I am talking about the weight that you put on, step by step, by making bad food choices.

So how can you even think that you can lose those pounds in three days? You are a human and not a machine. Even if you starve yourself, you cannot lose weight that fast because even the body needs time to understand there is no food coming in. When the body starts to recognize that, it starts attacking your stock of fat. But, at the beginning, it is water that you are losing, not fat.

And don't fall into WATER GAMES. They can vary every day. Again, that's just a number. The important things is to lose the fat. The smart thing is to take your time to lose the weight, so that you won't gain it back right away. Give your body time to mourn the lost pound or kilo so that it can let it go for good.

7. Don't Wait, Start Now (But Avoid Starting on Mondays).

When it comes to starting our new life or even a project, we always find excuses to not take the first step.

Don't procrastinate, as nothing is going to change tomorrow or in a week. Take the bull by its horns and start. As you know, the hardest part is starting, and then you can go step by step.

Why put off until tomorrow what you can do today??

STOP WAITING FOR THE SEASONS TO CHANGE THE VACATIONS TO BE OVER OR YOUR BANGS TO BE LONGER.

I would avoid starting any new lifestyle on a Monday. They are already a pain to go back to work, to school, or to daily life. Why do you want to add another stress to your Monday?

We wake up, already down and probably hungry. We try to stick to the chosen path, but by noon we are getting nervous, and by 4pm, we say, "I have been good all day. If I take a piece of chocolate, it won't kill me." By the evening, we think, "Well, I screwed up. I will start next Monday," and continue eating...

Don't become one of those who people who starts and stops a diet every Monday.

If we start on a Wednesday, for example, we are already in the middle of the week. We know the weekend is a few days away. Morale is higher. The chance of holding onto the new food life is greater.

8. Don't Eat Too Much Before Starting.

Every time we decide to control our food, we choose to eat as if there is no tomorrow the night before; our "last meal." It is usually composed of rubbish food, too much salt, too much sugar, and obviously too much crap. We think it is a good idea to stock food for the "hunger games." We feel full, but not completely satisfied.

The following morning, we wake up hungry. No kidding. All the sugar, carbs, and junk open up the appetite.

I can understand you doing this if you were starting a "diet." But do you remember what I have said? It is not a diet. It is a lifestyle.

You are not going to a starvation camp. You will just be eating healthier and making better choices.

Two

ARE YOU ON A SEEFOOD DIET: YOU SEE FOOD AND YOU EAT IT? (TIPS AND ADVICE TO CLEAN YOUR HOUSE AND SURROUNDINGS FROM TEMPTATION)

Before starting anything, you should clean your house and get rid of any unhelpful people around you.

By house, I mean your pantry, fridge, and freezer. I am sure you have already expired products and bad food choices sitting on your shelves and in your refrigerator. We will go through your stuff together to see what's good and what you should get rid of.

By unhelpful people, I mean the ones who won't support you on your journey. Don't say no. We all have those friends who push us to eat badly or who mock our new lifestyle. Who will bring you down and push you to eat crap?

9. Clean Your Pantry, Fridge, & Freezer—Get Rid of Bad Food.

Before starting, you need to rid your house of toxic food.

Open your fridge, pantry, and freezer. Throw away all the processed food and the refined chocolate bars that give you one minute of pleasure with a day of guilt.

I know it is harder when you have kids, but guess what? You are doing your children a favor. If they start eating healthy at an early age, they won't struggle like you did.

I am sure you know what to eliminate, but if you have any doubts, here is the golden rule:

GET RID OF EVERYTHING THAT HAS MORE THAN FIVE INGREDIENTS AND EVERYTHING WITH INGREDIENTS THAT YOU CANNOT PRONOUNCE.

Easy, right? So now you have no excuse.

Besides the fact that I want you to eat healthy, we know when we crave sugar, we first attack the cookies and chocolate, not the fruits. Or when we want salt, we attack the chips and cheese, not the vegetables. This is called the "seefood diet." We see, and we eat.

For example, if my fridge has veggies, fruits, and protein, I can only eat those. For a snack, I am not going to cook beef or a chicken. I simply open the fridge and attack the first thing that I see, so, in this case, my veggies. But if I have some pistachios or chocolate somewhere, I will attack them.

Believe me. I've had some serious nighttime sugar cravings. I was stalking around the house like a lioness, on the hunt for her next victim. After opening every drawer, every closet, or even looking in my purses for some candy or chocolate, I had to accept eating the apple in my fridge.

We might go to bed a bit frustrated, but in the morning, the craving will be gone. And you will be proud of yourself for having saved yourself from some empty calories.

10. Clean Your Closets—Get Rid of Your Skinny Clothes.

You need to rid your closet of the tight clothes.

You know, the pair of pants that you've kept for the last three years in the hopes of wearing them again—the pants that you try every other month, and they don't go higher than your hips?

Get rid of them. Why punish yourself? Don't forget: Fashion keeps changing every year. And your old clothes take up emotional and physical space in your life.

I went through my closet and either give away or stored away all of my tight clothes.

11. Clean Your House—Get Rid of Your Scale.

I don't want you to be obsessed with your scale. You are not walking around with your weight written on your forehead.

Don't forget: Each person has a different bone intensity. You can be thinner than someone else, but on the scale, the number will be higher.

Instead of the scale, I propose you should measure yourself. It will be more accurate and will allow you to clearly see differences in your weight and body.

12. Clean Your Friends—Get Rid of the Bad Seeds.

The same rules for cleaning your house apply to cleaning out those around you. I am not telling you to go without friends, but you need to be surrounded by people who will support you.

As of now, you know that I am traveling a lot and going out quite often. I must admit, in the beginning, it was stressful for me to incorporate my new-found lifestyle into my old lifestyle. I used to go all-or-nothing; go out seven days a week and then punish myself for two weeks.

So, I decided to find a balance and to go out without sacrificing my principles. Some friends were thrilled for me; some others started to judge me and tell me I was a party pooper. My mom calls those friends "bad seeds," and believe me, I had many. You know, the friend who always pushes you to eat or drink too much?

Tell your friends about your new life. If they accept it, great. Otherwise, keep your distance. You don't need negativity or toxic friends in your life.

I didn't erase the bad seeds from my life, but I started seeing them less. Instead, I have started seeing positive, encouraging people more.

With time, my new quest inspired most of my friends to also follow the healthy lifestyle.

Three

DOES A HEALTHY PANTRY INCLUDE WINE, CHOCOLATE, AND CHEESE?
(TIPS ABOUT FOOD SHOPPING)

13. Don't Ever Buy Groceries When You Are Hungry.

To start with, don't ever, ever go grocery shopping when you are hungry.

If I am hungry and go to the grocery store, I lose my mind. I buy every wrong choice that I crave, and I end up being the proud owner of aisle seven.

Naturally, when I arrive home, I eat all the wrong things first, and then I am too full to eat the right foods.

If you go to the grocery store with a full stomach, you are more rational, and you are better able to stick to your list. You buy whatever you need.

It is normal to think about buying food when we are hungry. Fight that instinct. Eat your meal and then go shopping.

If it helps you, make a shopping list in your hunger phase. It might give you some satisfaction. Read it again when you are satiated and edit out all the unnecessary garbage.

14. Avoid Buying Processed Food.

What is processed food? Right away, we think about frozen or ready meals. That's wrong. Any refined, flavored, or food modified from its natural state is a processed food.

So all the microwavable foods (or airplane food, as I call it), breakfast cereals, ketchup, and even soft drinks are processed food.

Processed food can contain a lot of sodium, fats, and sugars. So avoid as much as you can.

For example, if you buy chicken fingers and ketchup for your children, it is the worst meal you can feed them. And think about it:

IF CHICKENS DON'T HAVE ARMS, WHERE DO CHICKEN FINGERS COME FROM?!?!

Now, I also understand that we live in a fast-paced world and buying processed food is always the easy solution. Although I wouldn't advise you to do this, but if you really don't have time to cook and it is more convenient for you to buy processed food, remember read the nutrition labels very carefully.

15. Read the Nutrition Labels on Your Food

I know when you go shopping and start reading ingredients on the labels, there are so many words on the package that you don't even know what's in it.

BUYING YOUR FOOD WITHOUT READING THE LABEL IS LIKE EATING BLINDFOLDED.

Would you let yourself be blindfolded and fed (unless you are participating in Fear Factor)?

And don't forget, it can smell like chicken, look like chicken and taste like chicken, but if you don't read what it is, you won't know if it is chicken.

Do you remember our golden rule when you cleaned out your food at home? Get rid of everything with more than five ingredients and everything containing ingredients that you cannot pronounce. This rule applies to your shopping as well.

16. Beyond the Food Labels

Not buying processed food doesn't always save us from eating unhealthy.

Unfortunately, we don't know what exactly is in the products we buy. If you start reading labels, you will get confused at some point as there are so many: Antibiotic-free, cage-free, free range, grain-fed, grass-fed, healthy, hormone-free, GMO-free, gluten-free, and organic.

The bad news is that labels can lie, so the words on the packages don't necessarily tell you the truth. You were not there to see how they wrapped it, how they conserved it, and if the animal had a good life or not.

Remember the 2013 horse meat scandal in Europe? A famous brand, who claimed to sell beef ravioli and beef tortellini, was selling horse meat and other "undeclared meat." I don't know about you, but I prefer to know what I am eating!!!

So, what's the solution?

Use your logic when you shop. Obviously, you are not going to buy a chicken that has been radiated, and you should prefer to buy cage-free, pasture-fed chicken eggs rather than eggs that came from an unhappily, imprisoned chicken.

Buy organic as much as you can. We know if you buy organic, besides preserving our ecosystem, you will avoid ingesting chemicals, hormones, antibiotics and drugs in animal products, as well as avoid GMOs. And, it tastes better.

My mother makes fun of me because I buy everything organic. She lives in Turkey and buys everything fresh from the market. They are farm fresh, but she has no idea if they are organic.

Is she doing anything wrong? Absolutely not!!!

You are not obliged to buy everything organic. Your reason could be they are too expensive or you cannot find the products. Just make sure to wash your foods very well before eating them.

If you cannot buy organic food because of your budget or simply because you cannot find any, try to purchase farm fresh.

According to the EWG (Environmental Working Group), some fruits and vegetables are sprayed with pesticides more heavily than others. Here are the dirty dozen and clean fifteen:

The dirty dozen are the products that you should try buying organic. The list includes apples, celery, tomatoes, cucumbers, grapes, nectarines, peaches, potatoes, spinach, strawberries, blueberries, and sweet bell peppers. Green beans and kale are moving up on the most sprayed list as well.

The clean fifteen are the fruits and veggies that you can eat because they are not sprayed as heavily with pesticides. The list includes onions, avocado, sweet corn (watch for GMO), pineapple, mango, sweet peas, eggplant, cauliflower, asparagus, kiwi, cabbage, watermelon, grapefruit, sweet potatoes, and honeydew melon.

17. Don't Fall Into the 100-Calorie Snack Packs

Snack packs are sold in bulk of three or five 100-calorie packages. Besides the fact that they are "processed food," who seriously stops eating cookies after five little pieces?

I don't want you to end up saying, "100-calorie pack? Great, I need to open five little bags!!!" Basically, you think you are saving few calories, but you end up actually eating more.

We know sugar is a carb, and when we eat carbs, our body produces insulin, which causes us to crave more sugar. So, leave the snack packs at the grocery counter, and get a yogurt or fruit instead. And if you're dying for chocolate, buy real chocolate, and not a refined chocolate bar.

18. Your Fruits and Vegetables

This one is easy when you are at the grocery store: Stock up on fruits and vegetables.

Today, the new fashion is kale. You can find it at every grocery store and every restaurant. I wonder how we survived without it. Simply—with all the other vegetables. Kale is good as it is a leafy green, but you don't need to get obsessed about it and panic if you don't eat it during at least one meal of the day.

Any vegetable is good. The greener they are, more fiber they have.

Don't tell me, "But fruit has a lot of sugar." Believe me, it has less sugar than cookies, and it has more vitamins and fiber than any other sweet treat.

I encourage you to buy your fruits and vegetables in season and those which are particular to your region. They will be fresher. Every season has its own fruits and vegetables, as they grow according to the weather. If you live in New York, for example, strawberries won't grow in the winter months. If we crave them, we choose to buy strawberries from another warmer city. Just think: When you travel to Florida from New York, aren't you tired from the transport? Now think about those strawberries. Don't you think they will be tired from traveling from who knows where? That's why you should buy products that are locally grown as much as you can.

As I have mentioned before, try to buy them organic. It doesn't mean they have more nutrients or will make you lose weight faster, but they won't be covered heavily in fertilizers and pesticides.

My favorite fruit lately is watermelon. It stops my craving for sugar, and because it is full of water, I feel satiated.

19. Your Pasta, Grains, & Bread

Who doesn't love pasta and rice? I know I do.

Don't buy white pasta or rice. They are refined and processed. Their natural color is not white. I know some people say brown rice or whole wheat pasta has a different taste. I can understand that, but today, we have so many options.

We are lucky we don't need to eat full-on carb pasta. We have the option to buy vegetable pasta. I am not talking about the pasta with the vegetable flavor that just eases your conscience, but about the pasta made from actual vegetables. You can also buy a vegetable spiralizer and make a zucchini or squash pasta.

We know when we eat pasta that we don't care about the base, but about the sauce, so why not eat the healthy kind?

For rice, if you don't like brown rice, you have many other options such as quinoa or bulgur.

The same thing goes for bread. Read the label. Don't buy white processed bread. There are tons of different kinds of bread to choose from. Try them, taste them, and I am confident you will find your happiness in healthy choices.

20. *Your Animal Protein*

I believe we have to eat from all the food categories. So, go for it. Again, the easiest way is to choose organic because at least we know what the animals we're ingesting were fed.

Organic meat is, according to the USDA (United States Department of Agriculture), animals with access to the outdoors. They are raised on organic lands and fed with 100% certified organic food. They are not administered antibiotics or growth hormones. In other words, a "happy animal," which ate well, was cage-free and had daily massages. Their meat is a healthier choice, tastes better, and will make you happy.

When choosing meat, I try to eat more white meat because it is leaner. If you crave a filet mignon, then eat your filet mignon. Just don't do it every day of the week.

The same rule goes for fish. Try to eat more white fish because they have less fat. But again, it shouldn't stop you from eating tuna or salmon. I know tuna contains a high level of mercury, but it has a great amount of omega-3 fatty acids as well. Don't worry. As long as you don't eat tuna for every meal, you will survive.

Another polemic is salmon. I know wild salmon has a higher ratio of omego-3 to omega-6 fatty acids, and less incidence of disease than farmed salmon. The good news is, according to the Washington State Department of Health, they both have low levels of mercury, PCBs, and other contaminants. Today, it is harder to find wild salmon, and this shouldn't not stop us from eating it.

Even though farmed salmon contains less omegas, the ratio is still sufficient.

Stop obsessing and keep in mind the big picture. Soon, we are going to ask: Which movie was playing on the flight over that brought the salmon?!!!

So, enjoy your proteins, but as with everything, in moderation.

21. Your Herbs, Spices, & Condiments

Herbs and spices are the best and healthiest way to enhance your "unprocessed" food. Go crazy with your herbs. Thyme, rosemary, dill, coriander, parsley, sage... Each herb has a benefit and they are all delicious.

JUST BE CAREFUL. GARLIC AND HERBS ARE HEALTHY, BUT NOT GARLIC AND HERB POTATO CHIPS.

If you don't want to buy fresh herbs, buy them as spices (although they never taste the same as the real deal).

Condiments are essential as well to enhance the taste of your food. No need to say I am not talking about ketchup. It is everything but natural and contains high fructose corn syrup, which is unhealthy, very toxic, and acts like sugar. I am talking more about mustard, my favorite condiment. Besides its taste, mustard has a lot of benefits. Mustard seeds contain curcuminoids, which are great antioxidants, anti-inflammatory agents, and they aid in digestion. Mustard also contains AITC (Allyl Isothiocyanate), which is a colorless oil and is responsible for the pungent taste of mustard, horseradish, and wasabi. Studies have shown AITC to help inhibit the development of bladder cancer.

22. Fill Your Cart With Only What You Need

Now that we know to go shopping with a full stomach and what to put in our cart, we are ready. The next rule is not to over shop. Don't forget, you are not buying processed food, so your food does not contain preservatives to keep it for weeks in your fridge, freezer, or pantry.

So for the sake of being economical and to avoid eating perished food, buy just what you need.

To give you a visual aid, at the cash register, your cart should be half filled with salads, greens, and vegetables. The remaining should be fruits, grains, and protein.

If you feel like having a treat, get it, but don't go overboard.

How often you should shop? Well, it really depends on your daily life, but you should refresh your products at least once a week. Today, it is so easy to shop, even if we don't have time to go to the grocery store, because you can order everything online. Although, I personally love going grocery shopping, especially if it is a healthy store. First of all, I need to see, smell, and touch my fruits and vegetables, and every time I discover new products, it is like Christmas.

23. Buy a Food Processor/Blender/ Mixer

I am calling it a food processor, but you can buy a blender or a mixer. The important thing is to have one in your kitchen. Whether it's to make a smoothie, to prepare a salad dressing or any spread, a food processor is the perfect tool for your kitchen. You don't need to buy the latest and happening model. The basic one is fine. Even the Magic Bullet blenders are great.

With our busy lives, having a food processor cuts the time it takes to prepare our meals in half. Instead of trying to mix for an hour, by simply pushing a button, our soup or spread is ready.

24. Buy a Mandoline

You are going to ask me, "What is that?" If you want to cut, slice, or even julienne foods quickly, it is the tool to use. Just be careful as it is very sharp.

Basically, instead of wasting your time playing with a knife, you use your mandoline.

Besides the food processor, it is the tool that I use the most in my kitchen.

25. Buy Fitting Clothes

Clothes shopping is like the food shopping. You should simply buy what you need and not go crazy.

In our previous steps, we cleaned our closets and made space for new things.

Now, I want to you to go out and buy clothes that fit you. Don't look at the sizes or labels. Start by buying a few essential pieces, like two pairs of pants (one fancy, one every day) and a few tops. Learn to mix and match. You can always use your own accessories to create more outfits.

Why buy just a few pieces? Because I know you will shed those extra pounds and will need to go shopping again very soon. I prefer you buy clothes step-by-step.

26. Buy a Measuring Tape—How to Measure Yourself

I know that we all want to see our progress, so you should get a measuring tape. If you don't have one, go and buy one.

On your first time, measure your waist (the narrowest part of your waist), your arms, and legs. You can measure every inch of your body, but it is a waste of time and not necessary. Record your numbers in your food journal or in your agenda.

I know you will feel the difference in your clothes, but if you are stuck on numbers, you can measure your waist once a week to see immediate results. Your waist is the first place you will start losing weight, with your legs and arms following.

Four

WHEN WAS YOUR LAST SNACCIDENT?
(TIPS AND ADVICE ON HOW TO COOK)

27. Cook With Love

You don't need to be a big chef to cook delicious meals. You can find easy and practical recipes everywhere—in magazines, on the internet, TV, etc.

Cooking should not be a burden, but a fun thing to do. Put on some music or catch up on a television show, and enjoy it. The most important ingredient when good cooking is love. If you cook with love, your food will taste better. Think about a restaurant where you ate and heard plates breaking or angry cooks. How was your food?

I've had the chance to eat at the Chef's Table in several restaurants, which means you eat in the kitchen and sip your wine with the chef while they cook and prepare the food for the restaurant. Every time, I was struck by the harmony and calm in the kitchen. Believe me, it doesn't look like Hell's Kitchen where Gordon Ramsay spends the service hour yelling.

I know cooking is relaxing for some people, while it is a nightmare for others. If it is difficult for you, start slowly. Baby steps.

My mom makes always fun of me because I even boil water with love. Why not start with that? Be amazed how little bubbles are coming up. Believe me, you'll be pretending to be the host of your own cooking show in no time.

Start your home cooking career today. Get an easy recipe, put in all the ingredients, including love. I know it will be a success.

28. Cook Your Meals in Advance. Don't Wait Until the Last Minute to Starve.

Another essential rule. We all live busy lives, where we don't have time for anything. So instead of eating a nice meal, we opt for a quicker option. It can be a bag of potato chips, which will open our appetite to perpetual snacking.

As you know, I am not a fan of microwave meals. But if you want to be ready, why not prepare your own meals in advance? At least, this time, you know what's in it.

INSTEAD OF DANGEROUS LAST MINUTE SOLUTIONS, PREPARE YOUR MEALS IN ADVANCE.

Most cooked food can stay in the fridge for three to four days; vegetables can stay a bit more if they are safely stored.

For example, buy a pack of quinoa (or any other grain) and cook it on Sunday. It cooks fast, and you can use it as a base during the week for breakfast, lunch, or dinner.

Now you have no excuses. Prepare your meals in advance so you don't order-in or eat junk.

29. Cook Without Oil. Add the Oil After.

When you cook, there's no need to add a lot of oil to give a taste or prevent the food from sticking to the pan. You can add the oil once it is cooked.

At high temperatures, the flavor of oil will disappear, and if you don't use the right oil, your food will be toxic. So, stop using oil.

I am sure you are wondering how to cook without or no oil. Well, first of all, you should limit frying your food, but if you want to sauté and stir fry it, use other liquids. It can be water, broth, or even lemon juice.

If you use a non-stick or stainless steel pan that is sizzling hot, the food won't stick to it. The essential thing is to keep moving your food while it is cooking.

You can, of course, steam your food as well. I know what you are thinking, "It is going to be tasteless." Not really if you add good spices.

If you are like me and not of fan of steaming your food, you can always bake food in the oven. Most foods can be baked in the oven, even French fries.

As you can see, it is possible to cook without oil, so leave it in the pantry or fridge and start cooking healthy.

30. Cook With Spices, Herbs, & Condiments Instead of Salt

Why add salt when you cook, when you can use herbs and condiments instead?

When I cook my protein, instead of salt, I add a lot of spices, which creates an explosion of flavors. Another trick is to rub mustard on your protein. Besides giving it a good taste, the mustard creates a light crust around the meat.

For my veggies, I use water, broth and/or lemon juice, and of course, my spices.

Even for pasta and rice, I never put in salt while cooking. Once it is ready, I will add the salt if needed. Sometimes I will use sauce to enhance the taste.

Besides making you bloated, salt is dangerous and can contribute to heart disease or high blood pressure.

Condiments and spices, on the contrary, are strong antioxidants that fight diseases.

By switching one bad habit, you can get healthier.

31. Don't Fry Your Food, Bake It.

First of all, fried food is not good for you. All that fat can only hurt you. But if you feel like having French fries, you can simply bake them.

Preheat your oven, put a baking sheet on the tray and put the food on top. You will have that extra crunchiness if you put your oven on a very high temperature or broil for the last minutes.

If you are craving the oil, I prefer you spray some when it is cooked, then deep fry it. It will always be healthier, and you can digest it more easily while still enjoying it.

I don't remember when I last prepared a fried food. I bake everything. It is always easier and makes less mess in my kitchen.

You should not forget that, with your new lifestyle, you are allowed to eat at a restaurant. So keep eating healthy home, and treat yourself once in a while with the fried food when you go out.

32. Use Cheese in Moderation.

Most of us love cheese, but we don't need to add it onto everything or in large quantities.

I get it. My dream is to live in a house of cheese, where I can make my way out by eating it, but I've learned how to control myself.

I noticed in the U.S. that when I look for a vegetable recipe, there is always cheese. Sometimes it seems it is a cheese recipe with some vegetables as decoration. Very healthy, right??? No kidding. The poor, simple broccoli complains that no one likes him, so his friend advises him to wear some cheese.

Even in France or in Switzerland, where cheese is a part of daily life, they don't use that much cheese on vegetable dishes.

Although cheese is delicious, let's not forget that it is full of fat, calories, and that it is addictive.

Try to be creative and use other ingredients to give taste to your protein, carb, or vegetable. You have so many options. Stop being lazy, be creative, and "cut the cheese."

33. Cheat With Your Salad Dressing.

Whenever I make a salad dressing, I always try to substitute the oil with water or vegetable broth. I add spices and condiments, such as mustard. If I want it to be creamy, I add avocado, which is a good source of fat. I blend everything. If you don't like avocado and you want a creamy dressing, add Greek yogurt instead of mayonnaise. It will do the trick.

Some people even add fruits in their dressing. This depends on your taste and palate, but once you try experimenting, you will see you don't need oil in your dressing.

If you really want, you can add a spoon of oil once the dressing is blended. It is imperative to measure it and not put the oil in freestyle!!!

If you don't have time or don't want to be bothered by preparing a salad dressing, you can buy ready-made ones. As usual, check the ingredients first.

Now, we want a big salad, so lots of dressing. Instead of emptying the bottle of dressing, first pour two teaspoons into a cup, add vinegar, lemon, and/or water to taste.

Cheat with it. Don't forget the taste is very pronounced so you won't lose the flavor. You will just make it lighter and in larger quantity.

34. Avoid the "Freestyle" Olive Oil.

I am Mediterranean, and I love olive oil. I used to put olive oil on everything freestyle, and I wondered why I didn't lose weight...

Measuring my olive oil quantity changed everything. Use a spoon to put your olive oil in your foods. Just to let you know, one teaspoon of olive oil is 40 calories, and one tablespoon of olive oil is 119 calories.

I am not asking you to count your calories, but come on. When you think 100g (3.5 oz.) of raw chicken is 114 calories, you start to open your eyes.

Use olive oil, but measure it or spray it.

35. Have Your Snacks Ready.

Like your meals, you need to have your snacks ready. I am not asking you to prepare fancy ones, but make sure you have yogurt, veggies, and fruits in your fridge.

An example of a healthy and effortless snack would be a smoothie. You can make it sweet or savory. Another healthy snack is hummus. If you don't have time to do it, you can always find good hummus at the market. Although, let's be honest, boiling water, adding chickpeas and/or beans, then passing through a food processor doesn't require a diploma from a culinary institute.

Basically, with your snacks ready, you won't have a "Snaccident."

A SNACCIDENT IS WHEN YOU EAT AN ENTIRE BOX OF CHOCOLATE, A WHOLE BAG OF POTATO CHIPS, AND AN ENTIRE PIZZA BY MISTAKE.

You can find some easy recipes in the last chapter.

36. Cheat With Your Pasta.

We have established that everybody loves pasta. Today, the new fashion is zucchini or squash spaghetti. We can even find ready-to-cook vegetable spaghetti without carbs. It is great if you want to substitute and lower your carb intake.

But let's be honest, sometimes we want to eat the real pasta. To start with, I advise staying away from refined white pasta. Another important fact is the quantity. Don't make enough to end starvation in the world. The average serving of pasta is 2oz. (roughly 60g), which is not a lot. So how do we satisfy our craving without gaining weight?? Simply by cheating with ourselves.

With the following tricks, your plate will look fuller. You will eat a lot, but instead of eating 6oz. of pure pasta and sauce, you will eat 2oz. of pasta with 4oz. of vegetables.

My sister taught me a trick. Instead of using spaghetti, she uses elbows. You know, those mini twisted kinds of pasta. In the U.S., it is the pasta for the mac 'n cheese. If you boil a portion of elbows, add cut vegetables (I love it with zucchini and tomato), and even add some cheese (I like it with feta cheese), you will have a huge portion. You can find the full recipe in the last chapter.

Now, you don't like elbows but want to eat spaghetti, then use this other trick. Use your portion of spaghetti and add zucchini and/or squash to the spaghetti. The portion looks bigger and it is healthier.

For the sauce, have fun with it. As usual, try to restrict the cheese quantity.

37. Make Your Dish Look Beautiful. Don't Forget, You Eat With Your Eyes First.

We've finished cooking, and it is time to plate our dish. Don't forget, **WE EAT WITH OUR EYES FIRST**.

If the food comes in a weird mixture, we are not attracted to eat it, so put some effort in and make your dish look attractive. Do you remember when you were asked to cook with love? Wouldn't it be a shame to plate with hate??

I'm not asking you to plate like you are a pro, although, it is so fun that you will get more creative with every dish. I'm just asking you to make an effort and to not throw the food on a plate as if you are in the school cafeteria.

Don't forget: A beautiful dish will be a delicious meal.
For the sauce, have fun with it. As usual, try to restrict the cheese quantity.

38. Use Smaller Plates So You Think You Ate More

Another oldie but goodie trick. We know it, but we never do it. Especially in the U.S. where big is better.

I think one of the greatest struggles with losing weight quantity control. Using small plates will help us to control our portions.

By simply using smaller plates, you can easily shed a few pounds.

Five

IF I CHEW MY FOOD REALLY SLOW, WILL I BURN MORE CALORIES? (TIPS ABOUT EATING MINDFULLY AT HOME)

39. Eat Sitting Down at a Table Without Distractions.

In our busy lives, we don't take our time to eat. We keep eating on-the-go without noticing what we put in our mouths. The result is we become hungry very quickly again. It always amazes me to see people walking down the street eating their breakfast, lunch, or dinner on-the-go...

So, what should we do? If you are with your family, it is easier because you all sit around the table and share a meal. By the way, why do you think the Mediterranean diet works? Because you eat with your loved ones and share your food.

If you don't have family around you, don't lose hope. The only thing you need is to take your time with food. First of all, sit down at a table to eat. Don't eat your meal standing up at the kitchen counter. Then, try not to play with your phone, your PC, or any other distraction. It is your time to enjoy every bite of your dish.

Most of the time, people think that I never eat home, being a socialite and all, but staying home and cooking is one of the great pleasures in my life. I love recreating dishes that I tasted at restaurants, and modify the recipes. For me, eating at home is a ceremony. I had difficulty giving up my phone at first while I was eating, then it became a game. If you put your phone on silent for the duration of your meal, when you are done, your phone is full of messages!

Don't worry: The world can survive without you for fifteen to thirty minutes, and think about all the updates you will have afterward.

On your next meal, I want you to try this out. Take your time, enjoy the food you cooked and plated with love.

40. Eat Slowly & Chew Your Food.

In my family, we have a motto: "Eat fast. Otherwise, you will starve."

Over the years, I've learned to pace myself. Don't get me wrong, if I am famished, I am capable of inhaling my food. I work on myself to calm the speed.

Eating slowly will reduce your quantity of food intake, is better for digestion, and makes you feel satiated faster. One reason is the effect quicker ingestion has on hormones. Our hormones tell us when we've had enough food while we are eating, but it takes time to occur. So, if we wolf our food down, our body doesn't have enough time to tell us that it's full. Scientists seem to agree that it takes about twenty minutes for the brain to send the message to your body to stop eating.

So, you know what you have to do. Take your time to eat. Also, let's not forget that we'll have more time to admire our cooking!

Again, the meal should be a pleasure, not a burden to get over with.

WE HAVE TO CHEW OUR FOOD, NOT INHALE IT.

Don't forget to chew your food. I am not going to ask you to do it thirty-two times, but if we chew well, we will be satisfied faster, absorb more ingredients, and not have any digestion problems.

When we chew, we transform large particles into smaller ones which are easier to digest. Chewing also sends signals to our body to start getting ready for digestion, like providing your mouth with more saliva to ease the digestion. And finally, the longer you chew, the longer it takes you to finish your food, and as we have discussed above, slow eating helps you to eat less.

And guess what? By simply taking your time to chew, you can maintain or shed weight.

41. Start With Salad or Fruit to Make Yourself Feel Full.

Salads and fruits have a lot of water. That's why you feel full after eating them. I know, it sounds weird to eat fruit as a main course, but it is a great trick. Same goes with salads, so if you are conventional, go ahead and start your meal with one. Or even better, a salad with fresh fruit.

The good news with salads is we have no other choice than to chew them, so it keeps us busy for a while. At some point, I was eating so many salads before my meals that my teeth started hurting.

If we start with salad or fruit, we already feel full and have less space to eat other dishes.

42. Don't Drink Water While You Eat. Drink After Your First Serving.

Water is beneficial. You have to drink a lot during the day, but not while you eat. There are several reasons. The main reason is that our body is composed of 60% water. This fluid helps our body to function, aids digestion, circulation and body temperature. If we are low on those fluids, the body functions poorly.

Water helps our skin to be clearer and our kidneys function properly, and drinking water makes us feel fuller, therefore eat less. Sometimes, when we think we are hungry, it is just that we are thirsty. That is one of the reasons why I suggest that you drink a glass of water if a craving strikes.

So, if it is so good and suppresses appetite, why shouldn't we drink during our meals? The reason is simple. Our stomachs need to keep a certain acidity level, which helps with digestion. When we drink water during a meal, it slows the process and can cause bloating and poor digestion.

The best solution is to drink before your meal, or if you are really thirsty, after your first serving.

43. Listen to Yourself. Do I Really Need a Second Serving?

Talking about the first serving, we always have a tendency to eat more than we need. This could be because we are eating too fast and our brains don't have time to send the message to our body that we are full, or we just think that we should eat more, in case there is no food later.

Instead of rushing to get a second serving, take your time and listen to yourself.

Do I really need a second serving or am I actually full? That little question will help us to control the quantity of our food intake.

44. Taste Your Food Before Adding Salt.

Back to my salt issue. I see a lot of you adding salt to your food, even before tasting it. What is the rush? The salt is not running away. How do you know if it needs it if you don't taste it first?

So, lose three to five minutes and taste your food before adding salt, which will make you bloat.

45. Avoid Eating Raw Veggies and Legumes at Night.

I know, I know. We are all unbreakable and nothing can disturb our digestion, but those famous salads that make us thinner can be a problem if we eat them at night. This is simply because they are harder to digest, especially as we get older.

When we eat raw vegetables and salads, we don't lose the heat-sensitive and water-soluble nutrients. However, the high dietary fiber content can be hard to digest. This can lead to stomach pain and gas. During the day, we have time to deal with gas, but at night, it can disturb our sleep.

To make it simpler, keep your salad for lunch when you have the daytime to digest, and choose cooked vegetables for your dinner. These are a few vegetables to avoid eating at night—cabbage and family, peppers, cucumbers, onions, radishes.

The same theory goes with legumes, such as beans, lentils or chickpeas. These legumes, high in fiber, can create gas, therefore bother us while we sleep.

Six

DO CALORIES COUNT WHEN EATING AT A RESTAURANT WHERE I DON'T ACTUALLY KNOW THE CALORIE COUNT?

(TIPS ABOUT EATING OUT)

47. Don't Order All Your Dishes at Once.

In the past, whenever I went to a restaurant, I thought that I should order all of my meal at once. This way of thinking changed when I lived in Milan and saw my friends ordering their food. First, they ordered their appetizers, then pasta if they felt like having it, and then, if they were still hungry, they'd order their main course. I think this is genius because you are there to enjoy your time. I thought ordering your meal step-by-step made so much sense because if I am full in the middle, I can stop ordering or skip a dish.

So here is my advice to you: When you are out at a restaurant, you are not obliged to order all of your dishes from the get-go. Choose your appetizers to start with. Enjoy your appetizer and then see if you are hungry enough to order your entree.

Once you finish, think about what you want to do. Order another appetizer? Order the main dish anyway? Or would you rather share your main dish with someone?

The good news is that the restaurant and the kitchen are there if you want to order more.

If you order everything at once, you will feel obliged to eat everything, even if you are not hungry.

48. Always Start With a "Less Naughty" Dish.

Don't start your meal with a high fat, high calorie, high carb plate. It will open your appetite more. You can always order it as your main dish (if you are still famished).

Chose something like a salad or soup, or anything that is not too naughty and will save your calorie intake. With this trick, you can enjoy the main dish, or skip and attack the dessert.

49. Whatever You Order, Ask for the Dressing/Sauce on the Side.

Another essential tip is to ask for the dressing or sauce of your meals on the side. This is a great way to know that your food hasn't been simmered in the yummy but oily sauce.

Also, if you have it on the side, you will automatically eat less of it.

50. Share Your Food.

I am Mediterranean, so I love eating my food the tapas way. It helps me to eat and taste a bit of everything in smaller quantities.

To share your food, you don't need to be in a Mediterranean restaurant. At every restaurant, you can order an appetizer or entree to share. Obviously, this is easier for bigger groups, but if there are two of you, don't be scared to stay hungry.

You can always order more.

In my family, unfortunately, it is more than less. I think one of the main reasons why we struggle with weight is because they prefer to order everything on the menu, just in case. With most of my friends, we always share and I always end up eating less with them.

51. The Minute You Sit at the Table, Send the Bread Away.

This helps give you self-control. I know I don't have any self-control if I am hungry. So, if I am famished, I see the bread basket and butter looking at me... well, you know what happens.

Especially in restaurants where the service is slow, while you wait for your food, you keep eating the bread, and then you can't enjoy your meal.

On top of it all, bread is carb, so I finish my meal, leave the restaurant, and I am hungry an hour later. Basically, I pay for a three-course meal just to eat bread and butter... and I am still hungry!!

Go back to the basics of the "seefood diet." If you can't see the bread basket, you can't eat it. If you want to enjoy your meal, send the bread away.

52. How to Drink Alcohol.

People around me keep asking how I lost all that weight because they see me drink. I lost weight, but not my appetite for life.

I am not someone who drinks alone at home, but I like the occasional drink in social settings. My solution is easy.

THE GOLDEN RULE IS TO DRINK AT LEAST A GLASS OF WATER PER GLASS OF ALCOHOL.

My choices of alcohol are either bubbles or wine, because I play around with it.

If I drink hard liquor, I never mix with any juice.

For my wine and champagne, besides red wine, I always put ice in my drink. Believe me, it is not that I don't know wine or champagne, and if someone tells you the contrary, explain to them it is called a "piscine" (a "pool" in French), and that in St. Tropez, we drink that way.

Two birds with one stone: I take in less sugar, and I am cool. The other good news is that when the ice melts in your drink, you have more drink, so it helps you to drink less and be fresh for the following morning.

This doesn't mean that you should go out every night and drink like a fish. Once again, everything in moderation.

Seven

DO YOU CONSIDER PIZZA A VEGETABLE AND ICE CREAM A GLASS OF MILK? (TIPS ABOUT MAINTAINING AN APPETITE FOR LIFE)

53. Nat's Plate

I am not going to give percentages of the food you can eat.

Nat's perfect plate would be: For your portion of protein or grains, you should eat double the amount of vegetables. You want to use oils and dairy? Do it in moderation. Concerning fruits, eat them to cut your cravings for sugar or as snacks.

I am not asking you to become a vegetarian. I want you to eat a bit of everything. Just know that vegetables make any dish healthier.

Just in case you need clarity, a pizza is not a vegetable and ice cream is not a glass of milk.

54. Workout

Exercising is a major step on your road to a healthy life. It can help you to get in shape, but don't think it will be your only solution to losing weight.

I want you to have in mind that the more you exercise, the more your appetite will open. Those quick snacks will be helpful for those times.

The first thing is to find the workout which is convenient for you, and do it correctly. I have spent two desperate years doing an hour of cardio five days a week followed by weight training and Pilates. I was fit, but still fat because I wasn't doing it right. My trainer was a lovely lady, but she bulked me up instead of making me lean and thin.

Everything changed when I found a coach who was more suitable for me. My body transformed completely.

So, your number one task is to find the appropriate workout and trainer who suits you and to exercise correctly.

Once you start, you need to be consistent. You know how you brush your teeth every morning (at least I hope so)? Well, your workout routine should be the same. Whether you are planning to work out once, twice or five times a week, you should stick to it.

I prefer working out in the morning because it is when I have the most energy and I can start my day without guilt. One might also say: Workout in the morning, before your brain figures out what you are doing.

Be careful when you start exercising because you might get excited about it and set crazy objectives, such as working out every day. Don't go there. After week one, you will be fed up. If you have never regularly exercised, start with one or two days a week. Increase the frequency once you are ready to, not from the get-go.

I work out three times a week and I try to walk on the days that I don't exercise.

During my daily life, I never miss my sessions; it is like my religion. When I travel, I just enjoy life and don't run into hotel gyms. I am too busy having fun. Again, life is all about balance.

Now, if you are going to tell me, "I don't have time," it is probably true, but you can make time for it. You do have time to watch TV, right? Work out while you are watching television. You don't need to be in a gym to exercise. Or when you have to go between two meetings, walk instead of taking a subway. No time? Walk home.

There are no excuses; so less talking, more moving your body.

55. Have One Fast/Rest Day Per Week. 600 Calories.

First of all, let's make it clear: **FASTING DOESN'T MEAN EATING FAST FOOD.**

Fasting is staying without food and/or drink for a certain amount of time.

Once a week, you should clean your body by fasting or having a rest day. I don't advise you do it on a Sunday when you don't have to run anywhere, you have a lot of free time, or are with your family. Choose a day where you are very busy; when you literally have no time to eat.

If you are hardcore, go with fasting. By fasting, I mean spend your day with no solid food, just teas and juices, and if you want, a yogurt. And don't you think you can spend the day drinking sodas...

If this seems impossible, no worries, you can do a rest day, which is a 600-calorie day. Obviously, you won't take your 600 calories from a double bacon cheeseburger. You can find recipes at the end of this book.

If even this seems hard, start with few steps, like try skipping a meal once a week. Fasting even for a short period helps you to clean your body. Intermittent fasting allows the body to use fat as its primary source of energy instead of sugar. Fasting also gives our digestive systems a rest. Another advantage of intermitted fasting is to understand what real hunger is. If we eat every four hours, we don't understand the feeling of hunger. If we don't eat for twelve or twenty-four hours, we get a better idea of what hunger is, therefore we know how to listen our bodies better.

Fasting also improves immune system function because it reduces free radical damage, regulates inflammatory conditions in the body, and staves off cancer cell formation.

Be careful, though. If you skip a meal, don't eat two meals at the next one.

56. No-No for Soda. Drink Water Instead.

All those sodas you drink, even the zero calorie ones, are bad for you because they are full of sugar. Would you eat eleven big cubes of sugar? Well, if you drink a can of Coca-Cola, that is what you are doing!!! The same goes for all those sodas out there. And guess what? If you eat sugar, you will be hungry.

Instead, drink water!!!! It will first clean your body from toxins, and also helps you suppress your cravings. You think it has no taste, and it is annoying? Add some lemon in it or even fruit. Still annoying? Drink homemade iced tea (not the store bought that also has a ton of sugar), and try to limit the sugar you put in it. Yes, even if it is Splenda.

If you want to lose weight, keep it off and be healthy, you need to drink a lot of water.

57. Be Careful With Quantities. You Can Eat Everything, but in Small Portions.

This life rule is important to me as I used to eat big quantities. It is essential to control your amounts.

Portion control is a key point on the road to losing weight successfully. When I say portion control, I am not asking you to eat two carrots and a cube of animal protein. I am talking about cutting the second and third servings out. Even when we eat fruits and vegetables, they should be portioned, especially when we eat out and they add oils, butter, and cheese to give a flavor.

As my father would say, "The excess is the enemy of the good."

Therefore, eat a bit of everything, but in smaller portions.

58. Sleep

Sleep is one of the biggest problems in our society. I am the first one with sleeping problems, especially since I started having a cell phone. If I open my eyes for two seconds even, I keep checking my phone (just in case I might've missed something), and of course, I cannot get back to sleep. Does this sound like you? For some of you, the problem is not your phone, but your iPad or your computer in bed.

No wonder we cannot sleep. So why don't we get rid of all those things while we sleep. I found my solution. I leave my phone outside of the bedroom. It was hard for the first few days. I even went to the living room a few times to check my phone, but with time, I got used to it.

Sleeping is important for you to lose weight. Even if you do everything right but don't sleep enough, you won't lose weight. The reason is simple: Your body is so tired that it holds onto the weight to survive.

59. Listen to Your Body to Know When You Are Hungry.

Most of the time, when we think we are hungry, we are not. It is the idea of eating that attracts us.

I want you to think. When you say, "I am hungry," are you starved or you are simply bored and you want to fill up your feelings with food? I just don't want you to be hangry. "Hangry" is when you are angry because you are hungry.

You know your body, so when you have this feeling, check it out and ask yourself questions before eating.

For example, as I have mentioned before, don't feel obliged to eat breakfast if you are not hungry in the morning. I am normally not hungry in the mornings. When on vacation, I am. Maybe that's because I don't have to rush to my day, so I have more time to think about food. Is it real hunger? Or simply having too much time on my hands?

Another example is when you feel like nibbling on something because it is the weekend and you played couch potato all day. You are not hungry. You just had a huge lunch. You are just bored.

60. You Need to Eat and Vary Your Food to Lose Weight.

Common sense is that if I don't eat, I will lose weight, right? The answer is yes and no. Sure, you will lose a little weight if you do fast for a period, but the minute you start eating, you will gain all that weight back. So, starving yourself is not the solution.

Don't get me wrong, I fast yearly for two weeks. I am losing some weight, but my primary purpose is to detox my body and mind, to reset myself. I also know that when I come back and start eating regularly, I will gain some weight.

As you can see, I don't spend my life fasting. It would be sad to restrict myself from all of the food. If you want to have a happy lifestyle, you need to eat and vary your food categories. Don't start eating only salads all day long. That won't help. Come on, if that theory was correct then WHY AREN'T COWS SKINNY?? THEY EAT SALAD ALL DAY LONG. The same goes for any food. I don't want you to be bored eating the same food, and I don't want you to feel limited.

61. Eat What You Really Crave.

You know when you want that chocolate and instead of eating it, you end up eating everything you can find BUT the chocolate? And in the end, you eat it anyway?

That's wrong!!! By now, you should understand your cravings. If you really crave chocolate, go for it.

Believe me, it's better than doing a fridge and pantry raid.

62. Eat Without Guilt.

When I used to spend my life dieting, I undoubtedly kept cheating on my diet, and I always felt guilty. Good news today is that you are not on a diet, but on a lifestyle. So, forget about the guilt, because you can eat everything. Just make the better choices and check out your quantities.

Even if you eat a piece of chocolate, do it with pride. Don't hide. We are humans and not machines, and it is inevitable that we will succumb to temptation.

So why waste your time feeling guilty and adding calories for nothing? It is always exciting to be bad. So stop hiding and eat your chocolate or potato chips with pride. Enjoy every bite of it.

You know what? When we don't hide it, it is not that exciting anymore, so next time, we might not even do it.

63. Reduce Your Food Intake Before a Party, Restaurant, or Holiday. Not After.

You have this fabulous party coming up. Or even better, you have vacations planned in two weeks. Typically, we always say, "I will start my diet after the holidays."

WRONG. Start your diet before the holidays and reduce your food intake before a party, so when you are at your dinner party, you have some "calorie credits".

Whether I am invited on a friend's boat in Sardinia or on ski vacation in the Alps with my friends, I always give myself two weeks prior to the vacation to bring my act together. I know it is going to be all partying with pasta in Sardinia, or cheese fondue and raclette in the Alps, and I don't want to sit at the table and not participate. So two weeks prior to the holidays, I start being extra careful with what I eat, to gain some "FOOD AND WINE CREDITS." As a result, I arrive to the destination slimmer and can enjoy my vacation fully.

It's always harder to make it happen after than before.

64. Don't Get Obsessed with Numbers (Clothes, Size, Weight).

Do you see people walking down the street with their weight written on their forehead and their clothes size written on their clothes? NO. So why are you obsessing with those numbers? Clothes sizes don't mean anything. I can fit in a 00 and size 6 pants from the same store. So am I a size 00 or a size six? Who cares? I just feel good about myself.

The same goes with your weight. Some people have bigger bones, so their weight will always be bigger than what they look like. STOP reading those articles where they say you are supposed to be this or that weight. It is just a number.

YOUR IDEAL WEIGHT AND SIZE IS THE IMAGE YOU SEE IN YOUR MIRROR THAT YOU LIKE.

I understand if you still didn't ditch your scale because it makes you feel a sense of control. First of all, I hope you are not obsessed with it, meaning you weigh yourself ten times a day—you know, when you wake up, after the first pee, after the first poop, etc...

If you are in need of seeing those numbers on your scale, always weigh yourself on the same one. The doctor's, the gym's scale, and yours will probably show different numbers.

Weigh yourself at the same time of the day and don't forget to do it the same way—naked or dressed. Your result would be more accurate.

65. Get Dressed in a Way Which Will Flatter You.

You need to wear clothes which flatter you. Don't wear a turtle-neck if you have huge boobs and a tummy. Instead, wear a V-neck so you are sexy and don't look like barbed wire. For example, I don't have those never ending skinny legs, so I wear more flare pants. It makes me look taller and much thinner than if I wear a miniskirt.

You should **EMPHASIZE YOUR ASSETS**. It drives me crazy when I see a beautiful woman who gets dressed wrong and looks much heavier than what they are.

My mom always told me to enhance whatever is hot on my body.

Of course, most of the sales associates will tell you, "You look fabulous." They don't care about you. They care about their commission on your purchase.

You have eyes. Try different types of clothes and you can see which are right for you.

66. 80/20 Rule: You Cannot Be Good All the Time.

You cannot be perfect 100% of the time. Live your life by the 80/20 rule: 80 % of the time, eat and live healthy, and keep 20% to play and be bad. In other words, if you spend your week working out and eating salads, cut yourself some slack and don't work out on the weekend. Instead, enjoy one or two nice dinners with friends, where you don't check where the salmon comes or if your food is fried.

Don't forget, life is about balance. If you enjoy life, you won't be tempted to go back to your bad habits. That's the secret to being happier and leaner.

67. Be Bad.

Don't only cheat, but be bad once in a while. It could be with food or with anything.

For example, do something crazy, like don't check your emails for a whole day. Another example is to play hooky and not go to work one day, not because you are sick, but just because you want to spend your day being lazy.

As you can see, we can cheat not only with food but also with our daily lives. This journey is not all about food.

68. Don't Stop Your life. Go Out, Travel, & Socialize.

When we start taking care of our health and weight, we think we cannot enjoy life. On the contrary, you should enjoy life more. To start with, this is our new lifestyle. We're done with keeping ourselves indoors and ruminating over three carrots. We have the tools and know-how to behave in a restaurant.

We are done with refusing dinner invitations from friends and family. It is time to enjoy life. It will make us happier physically and emotionally, but also, don't you want to show your new and upcoming figure to your friends? Or even inspire them with your new quest?

Go out, see friends, travel.

BEING HEALTHY MEANS FIRST BEING HAPPY.

69. *Smile & Laugh As Much As You Can*

People don't smile or laugh enough. When I walk down the street, I see a lot of sad people. I am not telling you to be a dumb-dumb, smiling non-stop, but find pleasure in little things. Smile more and you will make people around you happier. In turn, you will be happier.

My friend's five-year-old daughter was checking my pictures on the wall one day. She turned to me and said, "You always smile. Why?" I said, "Don't you think it is better than crying all the time?" I am HAPPY (between us, even if I am not happy, I manage to make fun of myself and be happy about it).

70. *BE HAPPY!*

I know, life doesn't make us happy sometimes. We can't always change things, but we can modify the way we react to events.

When my niece and nephew were little and cried, I would tell them, "I bet you cannot laugh while you cry." They were shocked by my statement, stopped crying, and tried smiling. Guess what? The crisis calmed down.

We are adults. If the kids can do it, we can do it as well. And if you have difficulty feeling happy, once again, fake it until you make it!

Eight

IF YOU ARE WHAT YOU EAT, CAN I BE A BON-VIVANT GIRL?

What is a bon-vivant girl? If we literally translate it from French, it means "someone who lives well." So, can you be a bon-vivant girl? YES!

You don't need to be depressed at home to lose weight. On the contrary, you need to go out, socialize, travel, and enjoy every minute of your life.

You don't need to live on three celery sticks and water to lose weight. You just need to know what you put in your mouth.

If you want to be happy, healthy and skinny, you need to be a bon-vivant girl.

Don't punish yourself because you have a few pounds to shed. Love them, accept them, and then get rid of them with your new lifestyle.

Everything starts with you and your attitude, so no more excuses. It's time to start your new life!!!

BON-VIVANT RECIPIES

HOW CAN HEALTHY RECIPES NOT TASTE LIKE CARDBOARD?

(DELICIOUS AND HEALTHY RECIPES THAT WON'T MAKE YOU FEEL LIKE YOU'RE EATING SAWDUST)

These are some recipes that I have collected from my mother, books, and restaurants over the years. I have transformed some and invented some others. Enjoy!!!

1. Detox Day Sample Dishes

RICE DAY

5oz (150g) whole grain rice (raw)

1 cup (200g) stewed fruits

1 cup (200g) vegetables

Boil the rice with triple amount of water. Divide it into 3 portions. You will eat one of the portions for each meal with your choice of fruits or vegetables.

Crucial: no salt, no oil

FRUIT OR VEGETABLE DAY

3lb (1.5 kg) fruits OR vegetables

Divide your fruits or vegetables into 3-4 portions and eat only that during the whole day

Crucial: no salt, no oil

2. Salad Dressings

AVOCADO SALAD DRESSING

1 medium avocado
1 tsp mustard
1 tsp lemon juice or vinegar
1 cup (240 ml) water or vegetable broth
Fresh herbs
1 tsp olive oil
Salt and pepper

Blend all ingredients until you have a green colored sauce. You can add more water or lemon if it is too thick, or less water and make a dip. This sauce can stay up to 4 days in your fridge.

You can also use less liquid and use this recipe as a dip.

Variations:
I vary this dressing by replacing the mustard with wasabi, salt with 1 tsp of low sodium soy sauce, and use basil as herbs. Instead of only olive oil, I prefer 2 tsp of olive oil and 1 tsp of sesame oil. It gives an Asian version.

You can play with it until you find what you like.

TAHINI SALAD DRESSING

1 tsp of tahini (sesame paste)
1 lemon
½ cup (120 ml) of water
Salt, pepper, sumac*
1 tsp of olive oil

First, blend everything except the olive oil. Taste it and add salt or pepper if needed.

Once it is ready, add the olive oil and blend again to obtain a creamy texture.

Depending on how liquid or solid you want your dressing, you can play with the quantities of lemon and water.

You can also use less liquid and use this recipe as a dip.

*In case you don't know what it is, sumac is a ground spice that has a deep red color and a tart lemon taste. It is used a lot in the Mediterranean countries.

3. Dip Ideas for Snacks

HUMMUS/BEAN/VEGETABLE SPREAD

1 can chickpeas
1 can northern beans
1 tsp tahini
1 lemon
1 garlic clove, minced
Salt, pepper, cumin

For this spread, you can use chickpeas or beans or, if you prefer, both. Boil them in water.

Blend them with tahini, lemon, garlic (if you like), and the condiments.

I add different seasonings every time, and if you want, you can add a vegetable like cooked broccoli in the blender.

You can eat this spread with vegetables, such as cucumbers, celery sticks, cherry tomatoes, etc.

TAHINI YOGURT

1 Greek yogurt (I like the brand TOTAL)
2 tsp of tahini
1 lemon
1 garlic clove (minced)
Salt, pepper

Mix all the ingredients in a bowl and stir until it has a creamy texture. You can add curry or cumin to vary the taste.

4. Vegetables

CAULIFLOWER BREAD

1 cauliflower head
½ cup (170g) cheese, parmesan or asiago
1 egg
Oregano (or any other dry herb that you like)
2 tsp chia seeds (my new obsession and an excellent source of protein)
Salt, pepper

Blend the cauliflower in a food processor until it has the consistency of couscous. Drain the extra water with a kitchen towel.

In a bowl, mix with the cheese, the egg, and the oregano. Add salt and pepper and, if you want, the chia seeds. Combine until the mixture holds.

Put a baking sheet on an oven tray and spread the mixture into small thin circles. The thinner it is, crispier it will be. The size of your circles depends on how big you want each bread.

Put it in a preheated oven at 350°F and cook it until crispy. You can conserve the extra bread in your freezer.

You can use this recipe to replace pizza dough.

Variations:
You can make this recipe with broccoli instead of cauliflower.

Little Tip: If you feel bloated and full of gas, instead of taking pills, take one tsp of cumin. I am not going to lie, it tastes like mud, but believe me, you will feel relieved very quickly.

ZUCCHINI AND LEEK MUFFINS

2 zucchini
2 leeks
1 egg
1 tsp whole wheat flour
1 tsp shredded parmesan cheese (or asiago)
5 or 6 fresh mint sprigs, chopped
Salt, pepper

In a bowl, use your mandoline slicer to julienne the zucchini and leeks. Add the other ingredients and mix.

Put the mixture in muffin cups. I use the normal size or the mini cups.

Preheat your oven to 350°F. Cook for 20–30 minutes.

You can use other fresh herbs, according to your taste.

Variations:
You can replace the zucchini and leek by any vegetable that you like.

My favorite variation is with cooked and drained spinach, chopped into small pieces. I don't use mint for the spinach, but I add 1 tsp of nutmeg and chili flakes to give a kick.

5. Protein

PROTEIN AND VEGETABLE MEATBALL

½lb (250 g) ground turkey

1 cup (225 g) spinach, cooked and drained

2 zucchinis

4-5 sundried tomatoes

1 small onion

Salt, pepper

Fresh herbs (mint or basil)

Chop the spinach, the zucchini, and the sundried tomatoes into small cubes. If you want to save time, use your mandolin for the zucchini and then cut it. Grate your onion. Mix everything in a bowl and make small meatballs.

You can cook it either on the stove or in the oven.

For cooking on the stove, spray a frying pan with oil and place on stove burner. Once the pan is hot, lower the heat and cook the meatballs.

For baking in the oven, put a baking sheet on an oven tray. Put the balls on it. Preheat the oven to 350°F and bake them. After 15 minutes, take meatballs out and turn them so they are evenly cooked.

Variations:

You can replace the protein of the recipe. For example, salmon goes well with leeks and zucchini.

Once you have the hang of it, you can play around with the ingredients.

CHICKEN SHAWARMA

For the chicken:
2 tsp fresh lemon juice
1 tsp curry
1 tsp cumin
Salt and pepper
1 tsp extra virgin olive oil
1 garlic glove, minced
½lb (250 g) skinless chicken breast, cut into strips

For the sauce, use the tahini yogurt recipe:
1 Greek yogurt (I like the brand TOTAL)
2 tsp tahini
1 lemon
1 garlic clove, minced
Salt, pepper

For the table:
2 pita breads
½ cup chopped lettuce
6 cherry tomatoes, cut in two (I like the multicolored ones.)

For the chicken, combine all the ingredients in a bowl. Mix well and let it rest for 20 minutes at room temperature.

For the sauce, mix all the ingredients in a bowl and stir until it has a creamy texture.

Heat your pan and cook the prepped chicken strips thoroughly.

In the meantime, warm your pita bread, and put the chopped lettuce and the cherry tomatoes on the bread.

Lay the chicken on top and drizzle the tahini sauce.

I always make extra tahini sauce and serve it next to the pita.

6. Grains

ELBOW PASTA WITH ZUCCHINI AND TOMATOES

60g (2 oz.) unrefined elbow pasta (whole wheat, quinoa, etc.)

2 zucchinis

1 tomato

1 oz. (30g) feta cheese

1 tsp vinegar or lemon

1 tsp olive oil

Chili pepper

While the pasta boils in water with no salt or oil, chop the zucchini and tomatoes into small dice. Crumble the feta and add to the vegetables.

Once your pasta is cooked, pour it into a bowl and add the rest of the ingredients. Add some vinegar or lemon, the olive oil, and the chili peppers.

Variations:
As usual, you can vary the ingredients, but keep the measurements. For example, you can use brown rice instead of the elbow pasta and eat it as a rice salad.

ZUCCHINI PASTA WITH AVOCADO PESTO

2 zucchini, spiralized
1 tsp olive oil
2 avocados
1 cup (25 g) fresh basil leaves, plucked off stems
1 garlic, minced
1 tsp pine nuts
4 tsp fresh lemon juice
1 tsp olive oil
Salt, pepper

Once the zucchini is spiralized, put it on paper towels to soak up the excess water.

In a food processor, add avocados, basil leaves, garlic, pine nuts, lemon juice, and sea salt and pulse until finely chopped.

Then, add the olive oil and blend until it has a creamy consistency.

In a pan, put a little olive oil and add the zucchini. Cook for about 1 to 2 minutes until tender.

Add zucchini noodles to a large bowl and add the avocado pesto. You can season it with salt and pepper and a little parmesan.

ABOUT THE BON-VIVANT GIRL

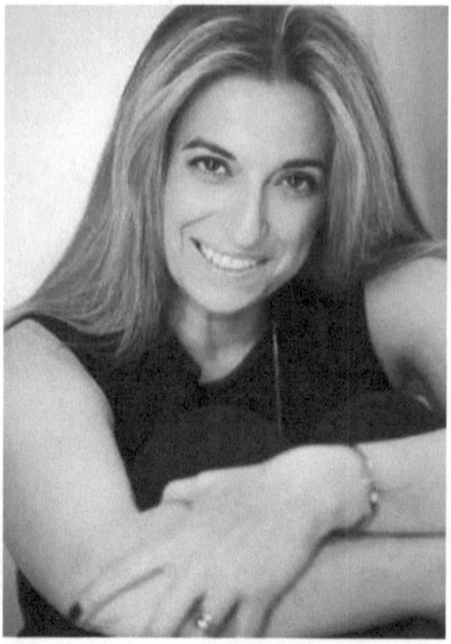

Nathalie Botros – the "Bon-Vivant Girl" – is a certified health coach and psychotherapist who teaches women how to lose weight and feel great without sacrificing their appetite and love for life. She is a world traveler with a big appetite for food and experiences. Nathalie was born in Lebanon, raised in Turkey, studied in Switzerland, played and worked in Italy before eventually landing in New York City. Nathalie started her first diet at fourteen years old as was the fashion in boarding school. From there it was a series of diets that varied depending on where she lived and what "little black dress of diets" was trendy. After years of being a serial dieter, Nathalie abandoned her "binge and purge" approach and embraced a life guided by balance, joy and living well. This new attitude put her on the road to a happy and healthy life... a bon-vivant life. To embrace the Bon-Vivant Girl's attitude for yourself, visit www.thebon-vivantgirl.com

Made in United States
Troutdale, OR
11/03/2026

56852547R00076